HEALTHY GUT SOLUTION

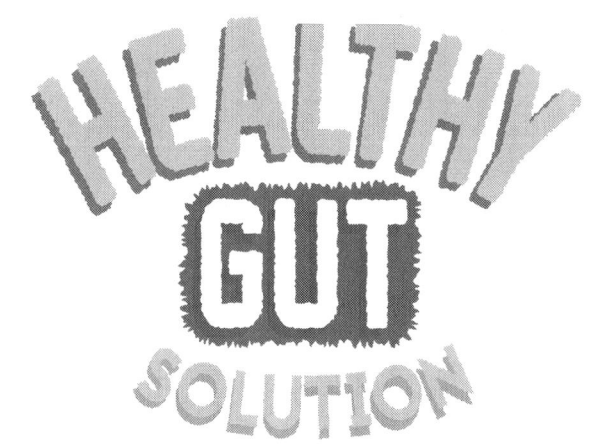

CARMA
books

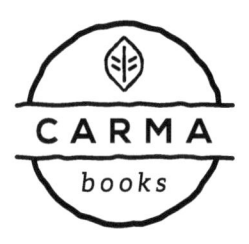

'A conscious approach to health & wellness'

carmabooks.com

You are invited to to join our **Free Book Club** mailing list. Sign up via our website to receive **special offers** and **free for a limited time** Health & Wellness eBooks!

HEALTHY GUT SOLUTION

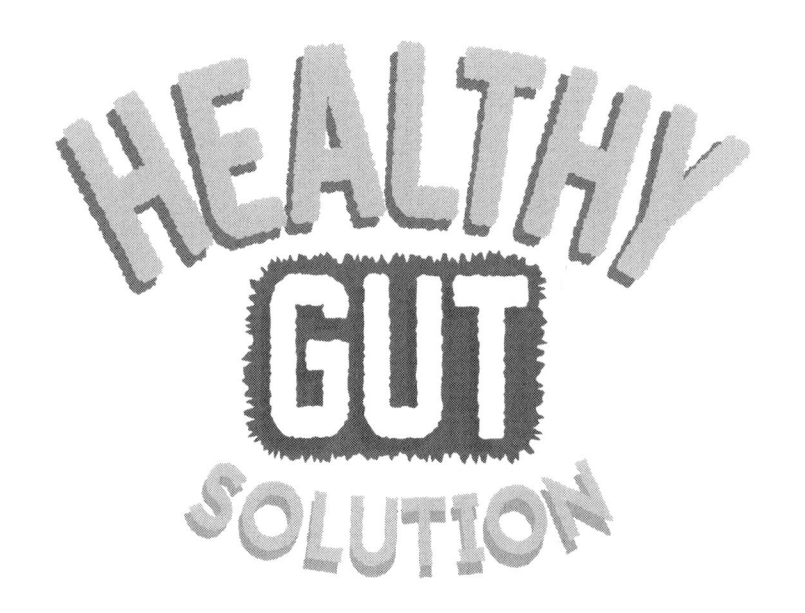

Carmen Reeves

Copyright © 2016 Carma Books

All rights reserved. No part of this publication may be reproduced, distributed, or transmitted in any form or by any means, including photocopying, recording, or other electronic or mechanical methods, without the prior written permission of the publisher.

Disclaimer

This book provides general information and extensive research regarding health and related subjects. The information provided in this book, and in any linked materials is for informational purposes only, and is not intended to be construed as medical advice. Speak with your physician or other healthcare professional before taking any nutritional or herbal supplements. There are no 'typical' results from the information provided - as individuals differ, the results will differ. Before considering any guidance from this book, please ensure you do not have any underlying health conditions which may interfere with the suggested healing methods. If the reader or any other person has a medical concern or pre-existing condition, he or she should consult with an appropriately licensed physician or healthcare professional. Never disregard professional medical advice or delay in seeking it because of something you have read in this book or in any linked materials. The reader assumes the risk and full responsibility for all actions, and the author or publisher will not be held liable for any loss or damage that may result from the information presented in this publication.

Carma Books
carmabooks.com

hello@carmabooks.com

CONTENTS

INTRODUCTION 8

CHAPTER 1
What is the gut, and how does it work? 12

Stomach 13
Small Intestine 13
Large Intestine/Colon 13
Heart and Blood Vessels 14
The Liver 14
Intestinal Flora/Gut Bacteria 15

CHAPTER 2
Why is a healthy gut so vital to our overall health? 16

Proteins 17
Fats 17
Carbohydrates 18
Dietary Fiber 18
Vitamins 19
Minerals 20

CHAPTER 3
What causes an unhealthy gut? 22

Lack of Nutrition 23
Stress 23

Eating Bad or Inflammatory Foods 24
Allergens 25
Lack of Exercise 25
Medications, Supplements and Drugs 26
Parasites 27
Common Signs or Symptoms of an Unhealthy Gut 27
Conditions Related to an Unhealthy Gut 28

CHAPTER 4
How can I promote good gut health? 32

Avoid Bad, Inflammatory Foods 33
Foods to Focus On 36
Herbs: Food as Medicine 42
Probiotics 53
Digestive Enzymes 57
What Else About Candida (Yeast)? 60
Lifestyle Tips 62

THANK YOU 70

A WORD FROM THE PUBLISHER 72

INTRODUCTION

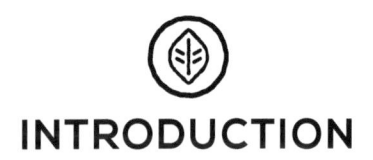

Thank you and congratulations on your purchase of *'Healthy Gut Solution – Healing Herbs and Clean Eating Guide for Optimal Digestive Health'*! This book will be a great first step on a path towards empowering your digestive health, an important building block for so many other assets of health and wellness.

Ever wonder why you struggle with certain symptoms and issues, reaching out for specific remedies or even medications—and seem to find no improvement? Do certain steps you take fail to work right away, whether digestive or related to other aspects of your health? Do you even go on healthy regimens or diets, in spite of your busy, hectic schedule, and still can't experience the changes in health and energy you'd hoped for?

An important thing to realize about health in general, is that *ALL* good health starts with a healthy gut: nutrition, whole foods, but most importantly, digestive function and improving that in and of itself. We live in a world where we take pills, supplements, and yes—even herbs and foods orally, in the hope to find relief. Most medicines and remedies are absorbed through our intestines, even the ones we take for intestinal health on its own.

If we don't focus on digestive health first and foremost, making it a #1 priority behind all good life changes we make, how are we to expect our bodies to properly assimilate and use the wellspring of natural remedies and nutrition that surround us? Makes sense, right? *All health and wellness starts with digestive health: and that is one of the underlying secrets to amazing health in its purest essence and power.*

It's become a clear worry in many developed areas of the world, that our current standards of nutrition and digestive care just aren't cutting it. Leaky gut syndrome, IBS, colitis, and many other digestive disorders are becoming more and more common, most likely as a result of potentially harmful foods and bad habits. Mainstream and affordable sources of both nourishing food and nutrition education can be adulterated with poor quality foods, filled with harmful additives, chemicals, and even allergens that we must take it upon ourselves to learn about on our own.

Certain modern medications, which can help with bigger issues, are no help either. Antibiotics, for example, can help save our lives from many acute illnesses and infections. But they have a very detrimental influence on our intestinal flora, and the natural populations of symbiotic bacteria thriving in our guts to help us with digestion.

To top that all off, we live in a busy, busy world. Many of us can be stressed out with wall-to-wall schedules and completely penned-in calendars, but we give little credence to having regular, healthy meals, or giving ourselves time to digest. We skip meals, eat in a hurry, or stop at gas stations or fast food places to get our fuel. This makes the problem of digestive health twice as problematic, but an even more urgent priority to focus on.

When we experience great levels of stress, what most of us don't realize is that our powers of digestion decrease even further. Stress increases cortisol levels in our bodies, which incite the "sympathetic nervous response," or the stressed "fight or flight" reaction. As a result, the more stressed out we feel, the less we actually absorb nutrients and much needed nourishment into our bodies!

It's not just about food itself, but many other factors that can deplete us. This will require not just a look at nutritional food and herbs—but at the very way we live our lives. I am an enormous proponent of food, it is true, with a passion for educating others about the virtues of finding nutrition from primarily plant sources. Avoiding a diet with too many animal products and harmful additives is a good start, but certain efforts and a sense of willpower is an equally important second step.

In this book, I will be happy to tell you all about how to take care of your digestive system and improve your health, involving natural remedies, tips, herbs, foods, science, and life changes that can be of immense help. Who knows—maybe some of the tips in this book will help with other health issues that have mystified you, and are somehow connected to your gut health.

These have all been of great help to me in my own process of strengthening my digestive stamina and power. Years ago, I discovered the reasons behind some of my own digestive health issues and other bodily struggles—as it turns out, I had a form of gluten sensitivity that when unnoticed, manifested as a number of confusing, frustrating symptoms.

I tried to help myself, using herbs, diet and other life changes, to make these symptoms go away. But it wasn't until I focused on the digestive aspect of things, researched some of the culprits behind my symptoms and removed gluten from my diet, that I started to feel great again and more in control. With some self-education and empowerment, I reclaimed my health. The energy and well-being I've experienced since the beginning of my gluten-free diet has been amazing and life-changing, along with other dietary and digestive health practices I have since adopted.

I hope that what I have experienced comes as an enormous benefit and asset to you, too, and you can find that path for you right here in this book. No doubt, you have probably heard of digestive issues such as candida, IBS and even acid reflux disease, or you have big questions and concerns of your own about your own experiences—and they have led you straight here.

Have doctors, medications and modern medicine not been the best help you can get so far? They can be, of course, when in a pinch. But take this book as a sign that it's time to change course, switch sails, and inform yourself instead of continuing to scramble through the dark. Yes, there is a reason you've stumbled upon *Healthy Gut Solution*, and it can be a good first step towards finding some answers... and relief. So, let's get started!

CHAPTER 1

What is the gut, and how does it work?

The gut is an informal term for our digestive system, which is made up primarily of the stomach, small and large intestines. It ties in the equally important functions of the kidneys, liver, pancreas, gall bladder, colon and even the heart, blood vessels and nerves. The gut can also be called the "GI tract," or gastro-intestinal tract.

Classically, when we think of the "gut," of course we think of our **stomach** or belly. While the gut often relates to digestion, we do not actually "digest" things in the stomach, as most people would think! It's true that food is broken down there, but most digestion actually happens in the **intestines** and the **colon**, especially. Food particles we eat are disassembled by stomach acids and bile, a secretion in the body created by the liver, but stored and released by the gall bladder.

Blood vessels run from all over our body to important sites attached to the lower intestines and colon, which absorb nutrients and transport them to the **liver**, and then all the various parts of the body that need it. Digestion involves a large network of organs in our bodies, some of which we might not associate with digestion, but it's important for us to understand the inter-connectedness of all these and how they lie at the very root of health itself.

Stomach

When we eat food, the first stop is the esophagus, the pipe-like organ that food goes down—and the next stop is the stomach. Again, this is just the beginning of digestion here, not where true digestion takes place. Food gets broken down here with the help of acids and "peptides" released by the stomach, and the strong muscle walls churn and shake food until it is sufficiently broken down, ready for transport to the small intestine.

Small Intestine

Here is where true digestion begins. Once food is broken down well enough, which typically takes a few hours, it becomes a more "fluid" substance called "chyme," and gets pushed through the pyloric sphincter into the duodenum or "portal" to the small intestine. The majority of all nutrients begin to be extracted here, most notably fats, proteins, and carbohydrates at this stage, along with the bulk of vitamins and minerals we all need. The pancreas at this point begins to release more digestive enzymes to aid with assimilation of nutrition, mostly alkaline ones, to balance out the intensity of the stomach acids.

Large Intestine/Colon

Digestion is finally finished off by the large intestines

and the colon, before food becomes a waste product. Water is extracted here, along with the remainder of vital minerals and vitamins that the small intestine might have missed: specifically vitamins K and B12, sodium, magnesium, riboflavin and thiamine. Digestion is not as strong during this stage, but intestinal flora and bacteria become a very important part of the process. At last, the remaining waste is pushed down into the colon for final absorption, then to the rectum to be passed out in elimination.

Heart and Blood Vessels

"Wrong system!" you might say. But actually, blood vessels are a vital transport of digested nutrients to the places in the body that need ii most, and thus make it a big part of the digestive system. In fact, the largest artery in the body, the "aorta," connects straight into the small intestine and is the largest distributor of nourishment throughout the body, via the pumping of the heart.

Another vessel, called the "portal vein," connects to the walls of the small intestine and brings it straight up into the next vital digestive organ: the liver.

The Liver

You could almost call the liver the "boss" or director of the digestive system. All beginning components of digestion (stomach, small intestine, liver, and blood vessels) end up here, for decision and process by this incredibly vital organ. Every nutrient imaginable is stored away, from fats and carbohydrates to vitamins and minerals, for determination of use by the liver.

Furthermore, "detoxification" happens in the liver as well, which is really a sorting process of both good and bad that has been absorbed and transported by the blood vessels straight from the intestines. Nutrients and toxins together come here and are further broken down and allocated. Of course, the liver keeps the good stuff, which is used through the body's metabolism, while exporting the bad stuff through various means, such as through the kidneys or lymphatic systems.

Intestinal Flora/Gut Bacteria

The human body carries about 100 trillion microorganisms in its intestines, a number ten times greater than the total number of human cells in the body. Some are beginning to consider intestinal flora and helpful bacteria as its own organ, even if these are separate living things that dwell in each of our own gastro-intestinal tracts.

During the digestive process in the large intestine, the liquefied food (or "chyme") becomes mixed with gut flora. These bacteria help metabolize further nutrition through fermentation of the chyme, and can be instrumental in processing vitamin K, B12, calcium, magnesium, iron, and carbohydrates.

CHAPTER 2

Why is a healthy gut so vital to our overall health?

Nutrition contains the building-blocks to overall health. Every vitamin, mineral, or other nutrient absorbed through the gut has a purpose and use, no doubt for another completely different system in our bodies. As I have foreshadowed to you in my previous chapters, health and wellness starts in the gut: our gastro-intestinal tracts.

So why is a healthy gut so vital? No matter what you do for other parts of your body to make them healthier—whether that's losing weight, taking iron supplements, or even over-the-counter prescriptions—these measures will hardly have an effect, if your digestive system doesn't function well. Taking care of our digestive organs, in and of themselves, is of course ideal.

Certain foods, behaviors, or habits can have an impact on our digestive systems. As a result, they can then interfere with our overall health, if not assimilating our food properly and getting it where it needs to go. For starters, it's important for us to remember the many different nutrients we depend on to be absorbed through our guts, to strengthen and nourish the rest of our bodies. Without a healthy digestive system, our overall health could perish, if it didn't get exactly what it needs!

Proteins

These nutrients are made of amino-acids responsible for the energy our bodies feel and generate through metabolism, as well as the strength and structure of our bodies themselves. They are common in foods from plant sources including **vegetables, beans, legumes, nuts and seeds**, plus meat, dairy and eggs—but do keep in mind that you can find all of your dietary proteins (plus an abundance of nutrition) through heart-healthy plant sources, not exclusively animals.

In order for the most basic building block, protein, to be utilized well for the rest of your body—good digestion is absolutely necessary for strong muscles, organ tone and overall health.

Fats

Yes—fats. Some fats are good, and some fats are not so good. Along with proteins, fats serve somewhat of the same function, in producing energy and providing solid building blocks for the body itself: adding structure to hair, nails, skin, and other tissue. Preferable to animal fats, good fats are found in healthier, plentiful amounts in the plant world: **almonds, avocados, and coconuts** are to name a few of the front-runners.

Digestion needs to be in working order for good fats to be of any benefit. For example: if you are targeting a new diet high in Omega-3's and beneficial fatty acids, to reduce inflammation in the body, **can a diet really help you if you don't attend to the needs of your digestive system first?**

Carbohydrates

Carbohydrates are the most essential source of energy for the body, and are useful in the storage and release of energy, along with some structure in our bodies and DNA. Common sources of carbs are found in **plants, grains, sugars, starches and fruits**.

There is some controversy about carbs in the diet, but what's trumped all opinions to date is that carbs are absolutely crucial for the body's overall function. Release of energy from carbs is almost immediate with the sugars absorbed, and carbs (specifically complex vs. simple carbs) do provide a host of essential nutrients along with them—including fiber, which is pivotal to digestive function. Complex carbs are vital to the more long-term, sustained release of energy over time, while some simple carbs are the ones you need to watch out for as less healthy (with the exception of fiber-rich whole fruit—think *highly* processed carbs).

Dietary Fiber

Fiber is one of the most essential food aspects that are vital to digestive health exclusively. It has an almost "lubricating," soothing effect on the digestive tract, as well as serving to absorb foreign or irritating other objects that pass through the intestines. In fact, fiber is so important to the human diet because it is the only thing that absorbs a great deal of toxic bile released by the liver.

Without fiber, too much acidity and inflammation would harm the intestines. Fiber is also a vital dietary nutrient in giving form and health to stools, and is found in abundance in **whole wheat, bran, fresh fruit and dried fruit**, but the very best kind can be accessed in vegetables—especially **leafy greens**.

Vitamins

Let's just say that it's fats', proteins', and carbohydrates' responsibility to take care of the bigger stuff, like actually forming bodily tissue, DNA and energy. Vitamins handle the details. We don't need as many vitamins for health, but in small amounts, they are absolutely essential.

Vitamin A, containing retinol for example, helps with the health of our eyes and growth. Vitamin C enhances blood health and our immune systems. Vitamin E is an excellent antioxidant and aids in the body's process/storage of fats, as well as the nerves. The majority of vitamins needed in our diets are found through a plethora of **fruits and vegetables**.

Minerals

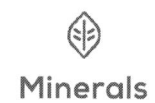

Similar to vitamins, minerals handle the remainder of the details. Iron, for example, can be found in **dark, leafy greens, beets and other vegetables**, and is vital to our immune systems and blood. Magnesium and potassium are pivotal for muscle health, and digestion too stemming from that—especially or the muscular integrity and function of the intestines. Calcium does the same for our bones, and can be found in high amounts from plant sources, including **greens, soybeans and sesame seeds**.

What happens when digestion can't provide us with what our bodies need?

When we don't get enough of the basic groups of nutrients above, it starts to show elsewhere, especially if the gut is not at its peak health. Lack of protein contributes to low energy levels, unhealthy skin or muscles, and even loss of hair. Lack of good fats can lead the way to precursors of inflammation, which then in turn create bigger problems like arthritis, cellular damage and cancer.

Lack of carbohydrates can have influence over energy levels and mental health, while vitamin deficiency invariably leads to severe health problems like scurvy, anemia, and even depression. An absence of various minerals, in conjunction with a digestive system that is not strong or healthy enough to process them, can show signs of damage and depletion to our bones, skin, immune systems, teeth, and blood.

It's a vicious cycle. When these things begin to happen, as a result digestive function worsens even further. For example, calcium (a mineral) is vital to digestive function itself in some ways, while no doubt proteins and fats help tone digestive organs themselves. Inability to process these nutrients thus makes the powers of the gut even weaker.

In the next couple chapters, we'll dive into the root of digestive issues—and how to nip them in the bud so you don't fall into that cycle. Food and nutrition, the root purpose of the digestive system itself, is important to the bigger picture. But it's important to know some of the precursors inherent to digestive dysfunction, which can involve many factors: avoiding certain foods, behaviors, and instead incorporating better, whole foods, vegetables, herbs, and lifestyle changes into your diet.

CHAPTER 3

What causes an unhealthy gut?

If we don't get the right nutrition, our whole state of health goes downhill. But what specifically leads to the state of an unhealthy gut in the first place, which then gives way to some of the symptoms of deteriorating health? The sources of this are many, and some of them can even be elusive and mysterious.

In our modern day and age, there are many potential harms surrounding us that our bodies didn't have to deal with so much in the past. It comes down to quite a long list of factors that can be difficult to prove, diagnose, or pinpoint without rigorous research, experimentation, and tinkering with your diet. Doctors can sometimes help, and nutritionists or dieticians can help us get through to the core of certain issues, but our main source of empowerment can be education—like the knowledge within this book, for example!

We all have different physiologies, and for each of us, there can be certain factors that have a greater impact on one person than another. To further dive into the contents of the chapter, I will go over, explain, and examine some of the most common factors that contribute to poor gut health. Perhaps some of these might resonate with or speak to you and your own struggles.

Lack of Nutrition

As outlined in Chapter 2, nutrition is the first step—and it may sound like a broken record, but it really cannot be emphasized enough. The foods we eat, both choosing and preparing them selectively, can be integral to good health, digestive or otherwise.

One of the biggest needs of the body for optimal digestive health is dietary fiber. Fiber is vital to digestion, as it mixes with digested food in a way that is healing to the intestines. In anyone struggling with gut problems, a look at fiber amounts in your food is incredibly critical. People who lack dietary fiber develop all sorts of bowel problems, starting with diarrhea and constipation. So lack of nutrition—but especially fiber—is incredibly detrimental and can lead to even greater imbalances over time.

Stress

Not many might realize it in the hustle-and-bustle of the modern world, but stress can be one of the biggest negative components of poor gut health. When we are constantly stressed on a day-to-day basis, cortisol levels increase, which send messages in the body to turn away the focus of metabolism on "rest-and-digest," and instead on "fight-or-flight": the stress response.

In simpler terms: when we're stressed, our bodies shut

off digestion, pumping blood instead to the brain and the senses. Decreasing stress levels can go hand-in-hand with a look at nutrition to turn your gut health completely around. Promoting a stress-free lifestyle, or at the very least minimizing stress in your life, can help you reclaim your health.

Eating Bad or Inflammatory Foods

Sadly, eating bad foods includes a wide category. Certain foods are delectable, comforting—but are they good for you in the long run? Overindulging in what we absolutely love is alright once in a while, but a balance is needed. Some people eat an excess of foods that, over time, wear away at gut health if no changes in diet are made, and which lead to even more disastrous health issues.

The more processed foods are, enriched with a wide variety of synthetic preservatives and acids, the more they disrupt gastro-intestinal health. Alcohol, coffee, dairy, carbonated drinks, gluten grains (if you are sensitive) and sugary/meaty foods are highly acidic, corrosive to the pH of your digestive tract and cause low-grade inflammation—inflammation easily overlooked by so many as "minor issues," until serious issues start coming on.

If you are experiencing symptoms of inflammation in other areas of the body, you may benefit from another one of my books: *Natural Anti-Inflammatory Remedies*

Allergens

Some of the biggest dietary turnarounds have been as the result of discovering one's allergens, and promptly removing them. Gluten and lactose sensitivity are the most common ones, but there are developing studies and observations on folks with legume (beans, peas, called "Favism") and nightshade (tomatoes, peppers, eggplants, potatoes) allergies. This is a new level of dietary need that is quickly coming to the forefront of modern nutrition, and certain allergies to certain foods have not been considered or taken seriously until now.

Take allergies into consideration, if you do suffer from digestive upset. This is a generally unexplored dimension of nutrition and digestive science, and *EVERY* person is different, no matter your race, culture, ancestry, or even background/place of living. To determine if you have allergens to certain foods, consider keeping a food diary and removing certain foods you suspect of being allergens systematically. Some exploration, including tests, into ancestral genetics can reveal a bit about what foods can set you off, and which ones don't.

Lack of Exercise

This can be a minimal, but overlooked, factor in digestive issues. Many of us forget that our digestive system is made up of many muscular organs. What do muscles need? Exercise! Hailing back to Chapter 1, our digestive system is thoroughly connected to our vascular system: blood vessels run along the walls of our intestines, colon, and up into our livers.

Think about it: if you lead a sedentary lifestyle and sit all day, circulation can be sluggish; what more, organs in the body can have a tendency to "settle," compact, or stagnate as the result of inactivity. Digestive-related issues like hemorrhoids can in part result from lack of exercise. Making sure you're being active gets your blood pumping, and brings fresh blood and oxygen to areas of your gut that could sorely need it.

Medications, Supplements, and Drugs

We know how uncomfortable digestive upset can be. Certain medications and pills, even though they are powerfully effective for certain other symptoms/health issues, can take away the vitality of the gut in a matter of no time. Antibiotics are a good example: while they are #1 on the front lines in fighting dangerous infections, they can throw off the entire microbiome of your large intestine. Vitamin supplements, which are meant to provide us with nutrition, can be made with protein-mimicking "excipients" that research has actually found to be harmful to the digestive health of some people.

Ever had a stomach cramp, and been prescribed over-the-counter anti-inflammatory NSAID's like Ibuprofen, or salicylic acid pills like Aspirin? Do you indulge in antacids if you get too much heartburn? If you are having gastric upset, taking pills that are doled out freely for uncomfortable symptoms might actually be doing more damage if you're not careful.

Parasites

While many of us living in the 1st World may believe that parasites are long behind us, unable to find a place or thrive in developed urban areas – this is not always the case. Even in clean and sanitary Western culture, parasites can take hold: as malicious bacteria, protozoans, insects, and more.

With a parasitic infection, the body will put on an inflammatory or immune attack in response, and digestive disorder will also inevitably be the result. Depending on the type of parasite, different symptoms will emerge – ranging from nausea and vomiting to abdominal pain, diarrhea, constipation, fever, and nutritional insufficiency.

If you suspect you have parasitic issues going on, make sure to narrow down the type of parasite you have according to its particular symptoms.

Common Signs or Symptoms of an Unhealthy Gut

Suspect that you could have gut health issues? The following provides a common list of symptoms that might indicate if you do. **This is not a list that**

diagnoses a disease, disorder, or illness of any sort. If you have some, many or all of these symptoms, feel free to contact your physician or healthcare provider if they are causing you great worry.

- Fatigue
- Constipation
- Diarrhea
- Alternating constipation/diarrhea
- Irregular bowel movements (from seldom to overly frequent)
- Discolored or misshapen stools
- Blood in stools
- Frequent pain, discomfort, or cramping
- Heartburn or high acidity
- Flatulence (especially foul-smelling)
- Incontinence
- Bloating
- Nausea
- Pale or sallow complexion
- Yellow complexion
- Unexplained weight gain, or weight loss

Conditions Related to an Unhealthy Gut

If an unhealthy gut persists long enough, imbalances may eventually give way to a systematic manifestation of more severe symptoms, in the form of a disease, disorder, or syndrome. Below are listed some of the major digestive disorders, what symptoms they might manifest, as well as the common origins that cause them.

If you suspect you have any of these, please seek medical attention for help, not just the advice of this book.

- *Chronic Constipation.* Symptoms of constipation persist for over 1-2 weeks or more, with infrequent defecation, suggesting an imbalance more so than a disease that should be addressed.

- *Chronic Diarrhea.* Symptoms of diarrhea persist for over 1-2 weeks or more, with overly frequent defecation, suggesting an imbalance but most likely, a viral infection that should be *immediately addressed.*

- *Induced Food Sensitivities.* Overindulgence of a certain food one has slight sensitivity to, coupled with poor health (esp. immune), worsens the sensitivity and can even make it manifest like an allergy. Food must be promptly omitted from diet.

- *IBS (Irritable Bowel Syndrome).* Also called "spastic colon," this is a manifestation of various digestive symptoms, most commonly diarrhea, constipation, or an alternation of the two, depending on diagnosis. Cause is often quite variable.

- *GERD (Gastro-Esophageal Reflux Disease).* Hyper-acidity of the stomach causes damage to the lining of the esophagus, usually due to a dysfunction of the lower esophageal sphincter, or barrier between the stomach and esophagus.

- *Candidiasis.* Overgrowth/infection of the *Candida albicans* fungus can affect the digestive system, most often after a course of antibiotics or as a result of lowered immune activity. This condition can be confused with other minor digestive disorders.

• ***Leaky Gut/Crohn's Disease.*** An Inflammatory Bowel Disease (IBD) brought about as the result of the immune system attacking cells in the gastro-intestinal tract. Can cause fever, bleeding, diarrhea and weight loss. Not an auto-immune disorder.

• ***Ulcers (Gastric/Duodenal).*** A break in the lining of the stomach or upper intestinal wall that causes severe discomfort, esophageal gas, vomiting, and sometimes weight loss and bleeding.

• ***Hemorrhoids.*** Swollen or inflamed vessels around the anus "prolapse," often caused by chronic constipation. Irritation, inflammation, and itching around the anus might occur, accompanied with rectal bleeding or bright red blood in stools.

• ***Colitis.*** A chronic or acute inflammation of the lower intestine and colon walls. When it includes ulcers, it can be called *Ulcerative Colitis*, a very severe condition similar to Crohn's. Symptoms are similar, including bleeding, weight loss, and severe abdominal pain.

• ***Diverticulosis.*** A condition of having "diverticula" in the colon, or worn away prolapses in weakened walls of the colon that create lesion-like mucosal outgrowths. Cramps, tenderness, and rectal bleeding are primary symptoms.

• ***Hepatitis.*** Inflammation of the liver commonly caused by a viral infection, but can also result from poor digestive health/behaviors: overconsumption of alcohol, and prescription drugs most notably.

• ***Cirrhosis.*** Chronic liver failure resulting from poor digestive health/behaviors: overconsumption of alcohol most notably. Cirrhosis can happen as the result of hepatitis and its common causes.

• ***Diabetes.*** This major illness, at an all-time high in America, starts with digestion and indirectly stems from it. As the result of a poor diet typically high in inflammatory foods, especially an excess of fatty animal foods (meat, eggs and dairy) and highly processed sugar, a better diet must be strictly regulated, or dire cardio-vascular consequences could be the result.

• *Small Intestinal Bacterial Overgrowth (SIBO).* A disorder of the digestive system involving the overgrowth of harmful bacterial populations over good. If chronic and ongoing, it can produce harmful antibodies that target and confusedly attack the body's own tissues, sometimes resulting in auto-immunity.

CHAPTER 4

How can I promote good gut health?

With the myriad factors we have to deal with in our everyday lives, focusing on good gut health might initially seem like a challenge. In some ways it is, as it requires us to avoid slipping into the comfortable trends or indulgences that can be so bad for us!

In truth, choices that contribute to our digestive health can be permeate every little thing we do: they are subtle, even hidden sometimes, making the source of our health issues tricky to figure out. They seem insignificant, small, or easy to overlook, but our answer to these choices can have huge consequences. What's vital to realize about our gut health, however, is that even those tiniest little choices can stack up quickly, creating a tower of problems that potentially crush our digestive powers. Once that tower gets knocked over, a failure in digestive health can have a domino effect on the entire body! All health starts with digestive health, and that cannot be emphasized enough.

That's why it's important to become conscious of all the little choices that can, instead, contribute to *BETTER* gut health, instead of the other way around. Just as the poor choices for our digestion can seem small and inconsequential, so can the good ones—just little choices we make throughout the day, for the better, can turn our entire state of health around.

In this chapter, we'll look at both choices: the little ones that can get the bad digestion happening, but also, the ones that can get things right. What's clear in this chapter is that there are so many MORE choices to make for good health, than bad. We'll touch upon the major factors or foods to avoid, and the foods (and herbs!) to embrace instead. The growing belief in nutrition and digestion today, is that food and herbs are "palliative remedies," or remedies that should come before we turn to bigger medicines, like pharmaceuticals, surgery, etc.

If we want to stop those other bigger issues from ever happening, we have to look at food—and gut health!—first. This involves a constant effort to make the little good choices, and to steer clear of the bad ones.

The Bad Choices

What should be steered clear of to balance and maintain excellent gut health? We'll dig into all the ins-and-outs, the "road map" if you will, of choices to navigate away from, and the ones you should navigate toward in this following section. Gut health can be simple, but having a guide before you can help you get started, without feeling too lost.

Avoid Bad, Inflammatory Foods
Perhaps the sneakiest of poor foods that creep their way into our diet, "inflammatory foods" are ones that are believed to create low-grade inflammation all

throughout the body, but first of all in the gut, of course. Often, this is due to food being too "caustic" or acidic for various reasons. Some of these foods are what you could call classic "junk food."

Inflammatory foods, if overindulged and made too rampant in certain diets, can lead to major diseases like cardiovascular disease, diabetes, and immune disorders like rheumatoid arthritis—and at the very worst, cancer. As a side effect, in can interfere with our body's ability to absorb and assimilate nutrition, thus impacting many other areas of our health as well.

The most common inflammatory foods are:
- *Trans fats* – the most undesirable fats you can eat. These are often found in animal and dairy products, but most often in foods with hydrogenated oils (many snacks and fried foods).

- *Saturated fats* – most of these are found in animal products, such as beef, chicken, pork, dairy and fried foods.

- *Refined or processed oils* – such as corn, soy, rapeseed, canola, peanut, and even olive, especially if cooked at high, smoking temperatures. These are the leading sources of trans fats, in fact, with animal products coming as a close second.

- *Refined sugars* – your classic, white sugar is a refined (and bleached!) sugar from sugarcane or sugar-beets, and should be avoided. Powdered falls into this category, too, along with the common containers of refined sugars: candy, baked sweets, and carbonated soda drinks.

- *Refined, processed and enriched flours* – like refined sugar, these flours are grain-based, bleached-white, and can often contain enrichments that are more harm than help to the intestinal tract.

- *Alcohol* – highly acidic and inflammatory, too much alcohol in the diet can create harm to gut health. Many alcohols, containing too much refined sugar, can make it three times as troublesome.

- *Grain/Gluten products* – gluten is a protein molecule found in most grains that can be formed into an even bigger, starchier protein as the result of baking. Gluten and other aspects of common grains, such as short-chain carbohydrates called FODMAPS, can cause a sensitivity among much of the population, along with digestive upset.

- *Processed foods of any kind* – any food that contains a high level of added chemicals, thickeners, preservatives, and enrichments is a processed food (not left in a near natural state). These include excipients, sulfates, MSG, food dyes, emulsifiers, and many other chemicals that can be disruptive to gut health.

The Good Choices

The good news about the good choices? There are many. So many categories, in fact, that you could say the good choices outnumber the bad. The true enemy to good digestion isn't really that there are so many more bad foods than good foods, but that the bad foods can just seem so good that they overwhelm the better part of our diet.

With just a little bit of effort, really, we can better dedicate the majority of our diets to those good foods instead, rather than letting the bad ones take hold—and which lead us to harsh digestive problems like IBS, colitis, and others. The key to good gut health isn't so much about eliminating every last delicious food in your diet to be healthy. It's more about being informed, conscious, and thoughtful about every food decision you make, even the smallest ones, to ensure that you are making more good choices than bad ones, for a start.

With time, making nothing but good choices—a perfect ideal we can all aim for—gets easier. But remember: beating yourself up over not eating perfectly will only create more stress in your life. Stress contributes to yet more digestive problems!

Foods to Focus On

Enough about the negative—focusing on these types of foods instead can be helpful and even healing to the digestive system, and give you a positive goal to shoot for.

Vegetables

Veggies of any shape, size, and color should be a high-priority for health, no matter what. Certain veggies, however, do have a more specific benefit to the digestive system, especially the higher in fiber they are. But really—any vegetable is good. Get in as many as you can throughout your day! 3-5 servings is typically the recommended daily intake, which equals to about 3-5 cups raw vegetables per serving.

***Leafy Greens*–** are especially high in fiber. The darker the greens, the better, meaning they're filled with many more nutrients beyond just fiber: like iron, potassium, and even calcium! Some examples are:

- Lettuces, Endives, and Escarole
- Kale/Collards
- Spinach
- Arugula
- Swiss Chard
- Beet Greens
- Broccoli and Cauliflower
- Cabbage
- Brussels Sprouts
- Turnip or Mustard Greens
- Chicory and Dandelion Greens

***Other Vegetables*–** while greens are the most notable and popular for digestive health, there are a variety of other vegetables that have high fiber content and their own influence on the gut. Some of these would be an amazing nutritional ally on your side too.

- *Beets* – not only have sufficient fiber, but the root has been hailed with detoxifying effects on the digestive tract and liver.
- *Alfalfa Sprouts* – fibrous and highly nutritious, with a beneficial effect on the colon, even with aiding in the removal of carcinogens.

- *Artichoke* – high in fiber, while bitter constituents stimulate appetite, digestion, and liver function.

- *Cucumbers* – high water content, combined with fiber, makes this a priority vegetable that cools and soothes the digestive tract. It has a widespread reputation for helping stabilize blood sugar levels in those with diabetes,

- *Squashes* – similar to cucumbers, most squashes (i.e. butternut, zucchini, spaghetti) are high in fiber, but also help regulate blood sugars.

- *Legumes* – beans and peas, including chickpeas and lentils, are fiber-high and nourishing to the digestive tract in those without legume allergies, or "Favism."

- *Celery* –both the stalks and seeds are very stimulating to digestion, detoxifying to the liver, and high in fiber, while helping the body eliminate excess proteins that could lead to gout.

- *Daikon Radish* – nutritious, detoxifying, and with a fair amount of fiber content.

Fruits

Fruits, along with vegetables, are the most beneficial building-block in a healthy diet, and a good choice in recovering gut health as well. Next to vegetables, a lot of fruits hold plenty of fiber, but also an abundance of other nutrition that creates a good choice for eating and getting your gut health back on track.

- *Raisins* – high in fiber, these also support the movements of digestion, from beginning to end.

- *Apples and Pears* – particularly if you leave on the

skins, these fruits are high in fiber. They can also have a cleansing, cooling effect on the intestines.

- *Raspberries* – high in fiber, rich in antioxidants.

- *Strawberries* – fiber is a good one here, while strawberries also happen to be one of the best sources of Vitamin C there is.

- *Cranberries* – have a decent amount of fiber, while their astringent action can be cleansing and healing to the intestines.

- *Melons* – such as watermelons, honeydews and cantaloupe. These are also cooling and cleansing, having an overall soothing effect on the digestive tract, but are also high in potassium—a nutrient that can aid in the muscular movements of the intestines.

- *Pineapple* – contains a compound called "bromelain," which encourages digestion and helps soothe inflammation of the gut.

- *Papaya* – contains "papain," helping in the digestion of proteins specifically.

- *Peaches and Apricots* – with the skins left intact, these fruits are high in fiber. Empirical study has also shown that peaches and apricots can help the body better digest and deal with inflammation due to food allergens the body accidentally ingests.

Whole Grains

Grains like bran, wheat, oats and rye are notoriously fiber-rich. However, if you have Celiac disease or gluten sensitivity of course, these types of grains are not your best bet. People who struggle with gluten should replace gluten grains with gluten-free variants, such as brown rice, quinoa or buckwheat, for example—and for various other reasons, gluten products can be more irritating and less healthy to the general population.

If you don't have to worry about allergens—grains are your friend! Focus on as many of these grains as you can, in tandem with a healthful daily helping of fruits, veggies, and plant proteins for balanced, complete meals. **Take note:** the more *WHOLE* the grains, the better, and some grain products even feature sprouted seeds of the grain, which help with digestibility of nutrients in other food—and help skip out on some of the possible irritability of digesting grains themselves.

Great Grains for Fiber
(Arranged top-to-bottom in fiber richness. Remember: the healthiest grains for fiber are found in whole grains, with sprouted grains being the very best!):

- Barley
- Rye
- Wheat (Spelt, Triticale, Kamut, Bulgur)

Going Gluten-Free, or Gluten-Sensitive? No problem.
The following are a number of grains that are notoriously and deliciously free of gluten. Even if you don't have a gluten sensitivity or Celiac disease, gluten products (especially in broken-down "floured," baked form) are still known to have a mildly irritating, inflammatory effect on the intestines. Consider omitting gluten grains from your diet, and instead replacing them with mostly gluten-absent grains like these, for overall better gut health.

- Oats (ensure you choose gluten-free oats)
- Buckwheat
- Teff
- Millet
- Corn
- Quinoa
- Amaranth
- Sorghum
- Wild, Brown, White, Black, and Red Rice

What else about food?

That's a good question. Is it enough that we simply focus on eating these foods? Or are there other things we should be taking into account, in conjunction with our food, as well?

An emphasis on *WHOLE* or "clean" untarnished foods is essential to getting the most mileage out of boosting your digestive health. For that very reason, I urge you to buy and consume fruits, vegetables, and grains that have been grown using **organic, sustainable practices** or which **have not been genetically modified**. Residual pesticides and herbicides can be incredibly detrimental to our digestive health, and a focus on heirloom varieties will ensure that the nutritional integrity of your food has not been tampered with, for the sake of something else.

Moreover—buy from a Farmer's Market, and make sure that your farmer uses sustainable practices. A farmer who grows vegetables on poor, nutrient-deficient soil is not doing you a nutritious favor, either, and their vegetables miss out on the very best of what you need. When buying grains too, avoid those that are **enriched or fortified**. The idea of added vitamins and minerals certainly is catchy, but frequently, the ways in which these "supplements" are added to foods only give you partial nutrition, in the form of caustic sprays that disrupt your digestive health more so than help you with adequate nutrition.

These are important elements to recall when making your food and dietary choices. But there's something else to consider—something else that is almost like food. It's almost like medicine, too. We'll explore it in the next section—healing herbs!

Herbs: Food as Medicine

The use of herbs is quickly becoming a popular therapy for all sorts of health problems. In my own mentality, herbs fall somewhere in between the spectrum of food and conventional medicines. Adding an herb or two makes for a lovely enhancement to your nutrition and diet changes, if you are careful and watchful of herb interactions.

Consider these following herbs, and explore which ones might be right for you. If you're overwhelmed by the selection—consult a trained herbalist or other skilled, professional practitioner with knowledge of herbal medicine. They can pair you up with the perfect herb(s) to meet your gut-healing needs, and inform you of the right dose/preparation. **It's smart to consult with**

an herbalist or doctor before starting use with any of these herbs, as they may interfere with other aspects of your health.

Bitters

Obviously, these herbs are called "bitters" because they are—well, bitter. As you'll read, bitters were historically added to alcohol quite often to make quaffs more digestible and palatable—a trick still used today. Without alcohol in the picture, bitters can be amazing for health… it's the whole meaning behind that overused phrase, "eat your bitter greens!"

When the tongue tastes something bitter, it messages the brain, and then immediately triggers the release of bile and stomach acids in preparation for enhanced, powerful digestion. Evolutionarily, our digestive systems learned to do this because the taste of something bitter often signaled that we might have just eaten a poison (poisons often manifest as bitter alkaloids). As a result, our gut immediately responds to the bitter taste with intensified strength, preparing itself to combat and rid the body of unwanted, hazardous plant matter. A funny connection, it's true—but it can only mean good things for the rest of our taste buds, and our digestion overall!

> • *Gentian (Gentiana lutea)* – This highly bitter herb once replaced the use of Hops in beer brewing, and was an additive to popular drinks, cocktails, and digestive tonics in the 1800's. Considered the most "classic" of all herbal digestive stimulants, Gentian root is in and of itself the very root of the term "bitters" used in modern drink-mixing liqueurs today. Avoid use if you suffer from a duodenal ulcer, or inflamma-

tion of the intestinal tract (colitis). Contraindicated in those with high blood pressure.

• *Yarrow (Achillea millefolium)* – Yarrow is also another excellent bitter, though it is not so much literally "bitter. It has a gentler and more pleasant, rosy, floral plant taste. At one time, Yarrow was also used to bitter beers, long before the advent of Hops. Avoid use if pregnant, on birth control or taking female hormone-replacement therapy.

• *Hops (Humulus lupulus)* – Today's modern-day bittering agent of beers, Hops totes a more citrus, pine, and fruity flavor that makes the bitter aspect much more delicious. The strobiles, or "cones," are also used in cooking and can make this herb an excellent appetite stimulant. Avoid use if pregnant, on birth control or taking female hormone-replacement therapy.

• *Wormwood (Artemisia absinthium)* – Wormwood was once used to flavor beers, along with the very telling drink in its scientific name—Absinthe. Obviously, large amounts of this herb are undesirable (unless you're looking for a wild time), but in small amounts, Wormwood can be the most powerful digestive bitter there is! Avoid use if pregnant, on birth control or taking female hormone-replacement therapy. Avoid internal use of essential oil.

• *Dandelion (Taraxacum officinale)* – Not exactly connected to ales and cocktails, Dandelion nevertheless has been hailed as a delicious, nutritious salad or cooked green. Its flavor is bitter and intense, with the root having especially prominent digestive properties—and detoxifying, liver cleansing effects to boot. You may also enjoy this nutritive green in the form of a soothing tea.

Carminatives

A little different from bitters, these herbs have a more separate function. Some of these help stimulate digestion and appetite, but another one of their wonderful uses is in calming digestive upset when it's taking place. Carminatives are "anti-spasmodic," meaning that they reduce cramping, pain, and spasms in the stomach and intestines by increasing blood flow.

Use these herbs for stomach upset, flatulence, or before and after meals. Some of these are culinary and good-tasting plants, too, which have been implemented into cuisines all around the world for those two very purposes: promoting gut health, and bringing out flavor.

> • *Angelica (Angelica archangelica)* – The stalks and seeds of this majestic European plant add a culinary flair and digestive enhancement to delicious foods. It demonstrates a warming and aromatic effect that helps remove cramping and gas especially. It is considered a danger to take while pregnant- please avoid use if you are, and if you are taking birth control or female hormone-replacement therapy.

> • *Thyme (Thymus vulgaris)* – A classic Mediterranean herb, Thyme is an ally to the gut in more ways than one. Not only does it dispel indigestion, cramping and gas, but it has been found effective in preventing nausea—a not so fun consequence of a severely disrupted gut. Avoid use of Thyme if you have an underactive thyroid or hypothyroidism, and

never ingest Thyme essential oils.

• *Spearmint/Peppermint (Mentha spicata/piperita)* – The origin of the "after-dinner mint" comes from mint's digestive properties. Spearmint is all-around excellent at taking the edge off stomach or intestinal upset, with Peppermint a close second. However, most herbalists will tell you to avoid Peppermint and use Spearmint in cases of acid indigestion, reflux, and heartburn. Never ingest Mint essential oils of any kind.

• *Fennel (Foenicularum vulgare)* – Ever see candied Fennel seeds at Asian restaurants? Similar to the dinner mint, Fennel is a valuable remedy for upset while being an appetite stimulant. Its licorice-like flavor makes it a tasty addition to foods and main dishes! Avoid use of Fennel if you are on birth control, are pregnant, or taking female hormone replacement.

• *Ginger (Zingiber officinale)* – Warm and piquant, Ginger root has been used to stimulate and aid with digestion starting with its ancient use in East Asia. The heat of this root helps allay cramping and discomfort of the gut, and to some extent, speeds up digestion while improving appetite. High doses not recommended for most as it can cause irritation in some, but especially the young under the age of 6. Some controversy over its use in pregnancy has erupted, but according to studies and statistics, it is relatively safe to use Ginger in infrequent, medicinal amounts in pregnancy. To play it safe, avoid its use.

• *Cinnamon (Cinnamomum zeylonicum)* – This popular spice has been on the front-lines with other herbs for indigestion specifically. It can also have a helpful hand in cramps, gas and stomach discomfort, but one of its most highly-regarded effects is its ability to promote appetite in those who lack it. Pregnant women should limit use to culinary amounts. Cinnamon essential oil can cause burning on skin, and never use it internally.

Antacids

The following herbs are the best "antacids" found in nature, and make up a small category. Nonetheless, the perfections of plant nutrition and nature combined have brought us these exceptional remedies for heartburn, acid indigestion, and even reflux to some extent.

• *Catnip (Nepeta cataria)* – Any good herbalist will immediately recommend Catnip in a heartbeat, at the mere mention of heartburn specifically. Try this cat-lover's favorite, which has a velvety and slightly minty flavor. On top of its ability to ease acidity, Catnip promotes digestion and relieves cramping, finishing off with a calming, soothing effect. Avoid use if pregnant, on birth control or hormone-replacement therapy. Some have reported allergies and gastro-intestinal upset.

• *Meadowsweet (Filipendula ulmaris)* – Turn to most herbal resources, and Meadowsweet pops up quite often as a powerful antacid remedy. Heartburn and some acid conditions could benefit from a try with this beautiful prairie plant, and empirical experience has observed its ability to be especially helpful to the healing of digestive ulcers. Meadowsweet also contains naturally-occurring amounts of salicylic acid, the same compounds found in Aspirin. Be cautious using herb with those having Aspirin sensitivities. Be cautious with those suffering asthma as well.

Digestive Tonics

Digestive tonics are just a bit different from these other categories, in that they don't deal too directly with symptoms of a struggling, unhealthy or temporarily uncomfortable gut. Rather, they strengthen and "tonify" the gut itself. Funnily enough, all these plants contain one important thing in common—fiber!

Fiber itself as a dietary nutrient is soothing and healing for the walls of the stomach, intestinal tract and colon, while helping regulate the consistency and health of stools, one of the more important markers of gut health (as icky as they are). On the other hand, these herbs are all rich in "mucilage," a damp but healing plant polysaccharide that removes inflammation and strengthens tissue in the GI tract, while also aiding with bowel regulation. Together with good amounts of fiber, consider these herbs for directly repairing and improving function of your gut overall.

- *Licorice (Glycyrrhiza glabra)* – This herb is popular, sweet, and incredibly healing. It is laxative when it needs to be, and an anti-inflammatory aid to any damage or irritation lining the gut. Furthermore—Licorice has a decidedly immune-empowering action, which can be helpful to those with Crohn's/Leaky Gut. Avoid use of pregnant, nursing, on estrogenic medicines, have high blood pressure or an auto-immune disease.

• *Marshmallow (Althea officinalis)* – Similar to Licorice, Marshmallow is overall regulating and stimulating, with slight immune enhancing properties. When used in higher doses, this plant leans more to the laxative side. Herbalists past and present have used it as a tonic and palliative care for digestive inflammations, like colitis. Be cautious taking this herb with important medications, as it can interfere with absorption.

• *Aloe Vera (Aloe barbadensis)* – Ever looked at the labels on soothing lotions or skin creams? How about using fresh aloe leaf gel on a burn? In small amounts, Aloe can be healing in the very same way to our gut, soothing inflammation and irritation just as it can help with dried, cracked skin, or speed the healing of burns. Aloe juice and gel holds no risks, but take caution using medicinal amounts of gel/juice with leaf mixed in, as it can be a powerful (and highly uncomfortable) laxative.

• *Plantain (Plantago major)* – No, this is not the banana-like fruit popular in Caribbean cuisine. Like all the herbs above, Plantain tonifies and soothes the gut. It can also regulate both diarrhea and constipation, bringing the body back into regularity over time. As an added virtue, it has been traditionally used for its excellent "drawing" and healing abilities to suck out infection and foreign substances in the gut, while closing wounds and ulcers. No dangers known, except rare instances of contact dermatitis.

• *Yellow Dock (Rumex crispus)* – In traditional herbal medicine specifically, Yellow Dock is irreplaceable.

It regulates both constipation and diarrhea, making it a powerful tonic for those suffering wide range of digestive ails, such as with IBS. It tones the colon, making it great for Colitis/Crohn's. Use has seen positive effects on those with highly acidic reflux, making it possibly helpful for GERD. Be cautious with its use, avoiding high amounts, and avoid use altogether if pregnant. Avoid administering to those with buckwheat allergies or high-oxalate issues.

• *Rhubarb (Rheum palmatum)* – Along with tasting great with strawberries in pie, Rhubarb is a powerful digestive tonic for those with fairly regular, healthy guts and who are simply seeking a little bit more "order" in their lives. This sour stem detoxifies, regulates, and strengthens, giving a laxative aid when constipation is especially intense. Use only stems, as remainder of plant is toxic. Avoid use in those with chronic digestive disorders like colitis and ulcers, and never use as a medicinal laxative for longer than 2 weeks.

Anti-Parasitics

Think you could be dealing with parasites? If confirmed by your doctor, implementing some of the following famously anti-parasitic botanicals could help get your gut healed and back in order.

When considering an anti-parasitic regimen of your very own, avoid going for "packet" cleanses or detoxes – these are meant to only be gentle modifiers that help with general digestive support and imbalance. They are not likely to help you with the detoxification process required to deter and remove parasites!

- *Black Walnut (Juglans nigra)* – The most popular herbal approach to parasites, the hull of this tree's large seed harms the exoskeletons of many common invaders (most notably tapeworms) and even killing them, thus preventing them from being healthy or successful.

- *Cloves (Syzygium aromaticum)* – This common household spice even as a powder helps change the overall environment of the digestive tract, to one that makes it harder for most parasites to thrive.

- *Garlic (Allium sativum)* – Similar to cloves, garlic's famous heat and pungency is very good at hampering parasites, preventing them from staying and proliferating successfully through your gut.

- *Wormwood (Artemesia absinthium)* – This herb simultaneously boosts the digestive system as a bitter, strengthening its own capabilities to dislodge parasites – while also having overwhelming and toxic compounds that affect the parasites themselves.

Tip: in combination with an anti-parasitic regimen using any of the above herbs, it's also very beneficial to up your dose or intake of probiotic supplements or foods. Increasing the amount of supportive microflora in your digestive tract can be a boost in deterring harmful, malicious types – and even larger parasitic threats besides just bacteria, like protozoa, amoeba, worms, and insects.

Further, opt for taking what is called "diatomaceous earth" **(ensure it is food grade)**, as well as activated charcoal along with the above herbs. Not only does the charcoal aid with detoxifying and absorbing the gut of unneeded debris, diatomaceous earth works similarly to Black Walnut: it destroys the exoskeletons of various parasites, either hampering or killing them.

Diatomaceous earth also helps "brush" away parasites from the walls of your digestive tract, while the charcoal will absorb waste (even parasitically laid eggs) before your body removes them!

Miscellaneous Herbs for Gut Health
It's hard to put any of the following herbs into the above categories, and yet they are still pretty important to take into account, when considering GI health. Take these healing plants into account when approaching various digestive issues, most particularly specialized, unique ones.

- *Evening Primose (Oenothera biennis)* – The seed pods of this beautiful, crepuscular flower are known to be high in Omega-3 fatty acids, very good fats and an integral part of maintaining inflammation in the digestive system. It acts like a digestive tonic, soothing and healing gut tissues, but has also been used traditionally for its observed activity on the "vagus nerve"—the largest nerve in our bodies, one that runs from the brain, to the heart, then to the stomach. Thus, Evening Primrose has been useful in treating digestive disorder as the result of nervous depression or anxiety. Avoid if pregnant or nursing.

- *Goldenseal (Hydrastis canadensis)* – Also a digestive tonic, Goldenseal is more known for its unmatchable antibiotic properties that make it an amazing remedy for certain digestive ailments. This rare plant contains berberine, a naturally occurring alkaloid which has scientifically shown itself to be one of the few antagonists against H. Pylori bacteria—a strain most likely to cause ulcers. Some forms of conventional medicine have even adopted Goldenseal as a front-line cure for most major ulcers. This plant is endangered, so be sparing with its use. Avoid use while pregnant or in those with high blood pressure, kidney disease, glaucoma, heart disease, diabetes, the very young and very old.

Probiotics

The microbiome of our bodies is incredibly important to digestion and gut health, though sometimes overlooked in more conventional medicine. Increased interest in the consumption, purchase, and even creation of cultured, good-bacteria is on the rise, as evidence-based medicines are starting to recognize that it plays a vital role in digestion. With that, of course, comes a mounting interest in cultured foods.

Probiotics are a great way of strengthening our gut flora, as eating high amounts of fermented foods introduces our current set of bacteria with completely new genetic material to fortify the current population. One can take probiotic pills (and I recommend doing so as a safeguard), but do ensure to also consume sources from whole, nutritious plant foods which can be much more natural and trustworthy. Many microbiota are of the genus *lactobacilli*, but there is arguably a wider range of helpful microorganisms than these. If there is a great need for probiotics and new gut bacteria in your digestive tract (i.e. antibiotics, digestive inflammation affecting microflora, yeast overgrowth, etc.), start with a high quality, non-dairy probiotic containing *lactobacillus* and *bifidobacterium* strains (30-50 billion CFU's), taking one capsule twice daily between meals. Follow by very gradually introducing an additional probiotic supplement containing *saccharomyces boulardii*, dosing in the same way.

The following section will explore the many varieties of healthful, plant-based fermented foods to further replenish and re-vitalize your own intestinal flora. No one's personal set of bacteria is the same as anyone else's, containing its own unique microbiome that is as peculiar and personally-distinctive as a human fingerprint!

• *Pickles/Fermented Vegetables* – You can purchase whole, cultured pickles at certain grocery stores and Farmer's Markets. Pickles don't only provide probiotics, but these same helpful bacteria have already taken the first major step of digestion FOR you: breaking down the tough cell walls of vegetable food matter. As a result, nutrition from fermented vegetables is incredibly easy to assimilate, and makes an uneasy gut have to work a lot less.

Make sure you check labels or talk to vendors, asking if pickles you purchase contain live cultures, as some ferments—especially common pickled cucumbers—can be pasteurized or filled with preservatives. If that is the case, it's unlikely that these products contain anything.

• *Kimchi* – This is an exclusively Korean-cuisine based version of pickles. Ingredients can be varying, but pickles are often spicy, featuring a hot pepper— along with radishes, onions, garlic, ginger, salt brine, Napa cabbage, and a shrimp or fish sauce.

Like standard America pickles, this makes the nutrients in the ferment immediately easier to digest, with readily absorbed nutrition. Kimchi is regarded somewhat as a garnish or topping to other foods as well, while it touts immune-stimulating capabilities and Omega-3's (from seafood). However, not all Kimchi's have fish sauce, so keep your options open for more plant-based versions!

• *Kombucha* – These popular brews are created using a colony (or mother, or "scoby") of bacteria and yeasts. The base of the ferment uses a caffeinated tea and some sugar, specifically a white sugar. The culture then "digests" the caffeine and the sugars, creating a pleasantly sour and effervescent beverage.

Those concerned with caffeine and sugar content can opt to make their own kombucha batches, and let them "digest" the sugar and caffeine a lot longer until it is no longer a concern. The longer kombucha ferments, the more sour it becomes, and it can turn into a raw vinegar if left too long. Many also love to create their own "flavors" of kombucha, crafting a brew and then adding juices that are then digested and broken down by the colony. Of course, the outputs to the fermentation is rich and probiotic-filled!

• *Sauerkraut* – Meaning "sour cabbage" in German, from where it hails, sauerkraut is basically fermented, pickled cabbage that has been pre-shredded before being brined. It is incredibly tasty, as many know, with sandwiches and meats—though some may not realize how healthy and tasty this condiment can be all on its own.

Like most common pickles, do check labels or speak with vendors about the sauerkraut you buy. Not all of it is automatically live cultured, as it is frequently pasteurized or preservative-laden.

• *Shrubs* – this is a very old probiotic food, but it is gaining popularity and favor of increasing proportions today, along with kombucha in a sort of "fermented beverage revival!"

Shrubs are made of chopped up fruit and herbs, steeped in raw, active-cultured apple cider or other vinegars, with fruit juices and raw honey. This is left to ferment, then quickly chilled. The result is a sparkling, fruity, and probiotic-rich beverage that can be sipped and enjoyed with more fruit juices or tonic water. This gives fermentation its own unique and exciting approach to fruits, instead of just vegetables.

• *Fire Ciders* – Fire Cider is a type of highly potent, medicinal, and culture-rich shrub. Hot pepper, garlic, ginger, horseradish, raw honey, and herbs of choice are placed in a jar, covered with raw apple cider vinegar, and left to ferment.

The result is a fiery, pungent, immune-stimulating, and cold-fighting medley that hits you square on the tongue, so brief sips are best. Not really known as an enjoyable beverage, it is more so regarded as an herbal-medicinal powerhouse to drink when sick— but it can push the body through viral infections, even helping on the digestive level. The probiotic aspect is often overlooked in this preparation, but it is most certainly there!

Digestive Enzymes

Of increasing interest and discussion in gut health today is the importance of digestive enzymes. These are an innate part of our physiology: being smaller chains of protein and amino acids, produced by our digestive system to assist with the breakdown and absorption of food.

Our bodies produce them on their own – but also get them from fruits, vegetables, and supplements. These are similar to probiotics in some ways, though digestive enzymes are not living beneficial bacteria. Rather, they are small chains of nutritive building blocks that our bodies produce and need to digest food and maintain health – all by turning larger complexes of nutrients into more easily absorbable, smaller, fluid components.

If our bodies produce them, however, then why do we need them sometimes through our diet or supplements? Unless you eat a predominantly good diet, rich in vegetables and fruits that don't get too overly processed or cooked, you might not be getting the digestive enzymes you need to get the very best nutrition potential.

As people age too, they lose the capacity more and more to produce sufficient digestive enzymes for optimum health. Of course, certain digestive disorders and other illnesses can impede digestive enzymes – all the more reason why it should be taken into consideration, much like probiotics!

Even if the above matters aren't what you are experiencing, lack of digestive enzymes could lead to certain very common symptoms as the result of insufficient digestion: including digestive disturbances, fatigue, headaches, thinning hair, brittle nails, dry skin, and larger issues such as thyroid disorder, joint pain, and reproductive dysfunction.

Sound familiar at all? Then it could be possible that digestive enzymes are something you need a little boost of in your life and gut health!

Certain natural enzymes are needed to digest particular foods, it has been found. You can get a wide array of naturally found enzymes in vegetables and fruits that are in their most whole, organic, and raw form possible.

A popular enzymatic tip: taking a tablespoon of raw apple cider vinegar 30 minutes before eating. This has been shown to help the body promote and produce its own digestive enzymes in preparation for meals!

How else to feel the benefits of enzymes? Here is a list of all the body, food, and supplemented-sourced digestive enzymes you can obtain by name. If you are otherwise not getting (or suspect you're not getting) enough enzymatic digestive action, you can seek out these enzymes in supplement form as well.

Make sure to discuss with your doctor first before taking digestive enzymes – and follow the label instructions depending on the supplement you purchase.

- *Alpha-Galactosidase* – helps assimilate the carbs found in legumes (beans, peas, peanuts)

- *Amylase* – breaks down starches

- *Cellulase* – processes fiber in vegetables, fruits, nuts, and grains (commonly known as "cellulose")

- *Glucoamylase* – assimilates sugars in grains ("malts" or "maltose")

- *Invertase* – helps process sucrose

- *Lactase* – helps process lactose, sugars found milk and dairy *(keeping in mind it's best to avoid dairy!)*

- *Lipase* – processes fats

- *Malt diastase* – breaks down carbohydrates (may contain gluten)

- *Protease* – disassembles proteins for better absorption

- *Peptidase* – can improve breakdown of casein from milk, and gluten from certain grains

What Else About Candida (Yeast)?

Candida overgrowth *(Candida albicans)* is a commonly overlooked condition that many experience as a result of a variety of causes, such as: an unhealthy digestive system, numerous courses of antibiotics throughout life, birth control pills, lowered immunity, poor diet, insulin resistance and diabetes, acidity and even stress. It occurs when candida, a naturally present fungus in the digestive system, is overproduced and can multiply throughout the body causing inflammation and poor health.

An acidic body over time can cause candida to become systemic, resulting in many generalized and confusing symptoms for sufferers, including: chronic fatigue, mood swings, depression, brain fog, strong sugar cravings, autoimmune flare-ups, digestive issues, skin and nail fungal infections, itchy ears, white coating on tongue, and recurring vaginal and urinary tract infections, to name just a few.

Along with an anti-inflammatory diet and probiotics, some naturally effective antifungal herbs to discourage candida growth include:

- *Pau d'Arco (Lapacho)* – a powerful antifungal tree bark imported from Paraguay, Brazil and Argentina, which inhibits the growth of candida and infections, and stimulates the bowels to cleanse the gut and expose candida yeast. Available in both capsule and tea form. *Do not take if pregnant, breastfeeding, at risk of blood thinning disorders or anticipating a forthcoming surgery.*

• *Olive Leaf Extract* – this popular herbal treatment strengthens your immune system to fight off unwanted candida species and intruders. It can also help stabilize blood sugar levels as fluctuations can feed candida overgrowth. Take smaller doses first, then increase to 2 (500mg) capsules 3 times daily with meals. *Do not take if pregnant, breastfeeding, diabetic, or taking blood pressure medication.*

• *Goldenseal (Hydrastis canadensis)* – its active ingredient, *berberine*, has been proven to inhibit the growth of candida and help support the immune system, ultimately strengthening your body's ability to fight off infections and yeast. Start low and slow and gradually increase dosage as per instructions on the bottle. *Be cautious that large quantities can irritate the liver. Do not take if pregnant or breastfeeding.*

You may experience candida die-off symptoms. Rapidly ridding candida can create a die-off reaction that temporarily releases metabolic by-products and toxins into the body. For this reason, professional guidance is recommended during this process with a practitioner experienced in treating candida. If you experience any of the following initial symptoms as a result of taking antifungals, this may be a result of candida leaving your body and will usually resolve within 10 days.

- Brain fog
- Headaches

- Fatigue
- Lower back ache
- Digestive distress such as gas, constipation or diarrhea
- Dizziness
- Sweating, chills and flu-like symptoms
- Skin breakouts

If die-off symptoms are severe, reduce the dosage of antifungals or stop altogether for a few days. Always start low and slow and gradually increase to the instructed dosage. When your symptoms have resolved, continue to take high quality probiotics and eat an anti-inflammatory, high fiber, low acid diet as outlined in this book, remembering to avoid low-fiber inflammatory foods that can ferment in the gut.

Lifestyle Tips

With approaching gut health, it can be much too easy to underestimate the very way we live our lives as part of the problem. Digestion can be at the very root cause of many ails—but at the even deeper root of digestion itself can be our decisions, attitudes, and lifestyle factors.

Those who think to themselves "these herbs and medicines aren't working!" or "no matter how nutritiously I eat, it always seems like I just stay in the same place," might need to look at the choices they are making that could be leading to bad digestive health and habits.

Even the smallest, most insignificant choices should be turned over and considered.

If digestion isn't happening in a great way for you, consider that there might be something mentally, emotionally, and even spiritually involved. Why am I eating these bad foods? Why don't I have the time to reconfigure my diet? Why don't I feel motivated to make a change? This following section will provide potential areas or methods to consider or alter, if the trail of your digestive issues is starting to run cold.

Alleviate Stress
Yes, care for the digestive system can merge into the realm of counseling at times. Some doctors and health practitioners will address stress with a patient or during a protocol as a very important and even physiological factor. Stress can creep into our lives for mental, emotional, and even spiritual reasons—and when our bodies can't cope, digestion is one of the first things to shut down, along with nervous and mental function.

The vagus nerve, which runs from our brains down to our hearts and digestive systems, plays a major role in digestion as it relates to the outside world and stimuli. During stressful times or even depression, the "fight or flight" response is triggered through this nerve, effectively making digestion a low priority and shutting it down. Someone who is in a constantly stressed out, anxious, or depressed state automatically has deprived, compromised gut function. As such, stress itself is imperative in studying how to get back to a healthy state, or everything else you do might just not work at all.

Here is an example: you work wall-to-wall hours trying to get by with your job. You're dealing with stressful co-workers, in an environment where you just cannot feel enlightened, no matter how hard you try. There's hardly a moment for meals, even when you do try to make them healthier and more wholesome. There are certainly some bowel issues going on or that are starting to show. While you do try to eat healthy, more often than not it just feels easier to grab something quick but unhealthy, and of much lesser quality. Perhaps in your spare time, you drink quite a bit for stress relief, or even smoke cigarettes.

Obviously, there are a lot of big problems here. It might be easy first to point out that this person eats poorly, drinks and smokes, and that they should change. But the real problem is stress: the underlying cause for this person turning to easier but less healthy outlets which only feed into a vicious cycle. This is an incredibly good reason why stress must be taken into consideration, no matter what.

If this person changed jobs to a place where they felt less stressed and more respected, they might feel happier and more light-hearted. They might then feel more motivated to take health into their own hands, choosing a *LOT* better foods, instead of eating junk or consuming substances as a release. If they worked less or tried to manage their hours, obviously, they would have more time to make better choices, and actually take time to think about what they're eating—instead of feeling rushed, rushed, rushed!

Stress would diminish, digestion would be restored, and good choices would be made. By including stress in the picture, you can follow the trail of your digestive issues to bigger issues in your life which you could take control of.

Exercise

Being active *CAN* alleviate stress, so you're really hitting two birds with one stone here. Consider exercise as a daily or weekly regimen, but also remember that your digestive system is made up largely of a number of powerful muscles, supplied by many oxygen- and blood-rich vessels.

Getting aerobic exercise might get your gut moving and healing in ways you never thought possible, especially if you are living a stagnant, sedentary lifestyle that fails to bring fresh supply where your body really needs it. Remember: blood vessels, too, are responsible for carrying nutrition around your body. Your heart also needs to be healthy in order to get nutrients, vitamins, minerals, and macronutrients to their proper places, and nothing helps your heart better than regular aerobic exercise!

Jogging, swimming, and even just walking a few miles a day can have enormous effects. Symptoms like constipation can be partially cleared up simply by changing your routine to a more active one. Even anaerobic exercise has its benefits too, like weightlifting, sit-ups, and other exercises. While it doesn't benefit the heart as powerfully, your digestive muscles are certainly moved around, strengthened, and toned to deal with digestion in a more dynamic way.

Yoga

Yoga is certainly exercise, it's true. It's also anaerobic, making it not as heart-healthy or rigorously impactful on digestive health in some ways. On the other hand, certain yoga stretches and practices *CAN* stimulate, activate, or help bring yet more blood to certain parts of the body. It can be argued that yoga, as an adjunct to or replacement of exercise, can be quite powerful all the same.

Consider or look up some of the following stretches or poses:

- *Half Moon Pose (Parivrtta Ardhachandrasana)* – tones the abdominal organs

- *Standing Splits (Urdhva Prasarita Eka Padasana)* – brings circulation to the abdominal organs

- *Revolved Side Angle Stretch (Parivrtta Parsvakonasana)* – this stretch involves a twist of the abdomen that "squeezes" abdominal organs, and involves gentle massage, which can help with digestive function.

- *Bound Lotus Posture (Baddha Padmasana)* – a forward bend that assists and speeds digestion and elimination.

Party Less!

For those who do like to let their hair down once in a while, it's a no-brainer that doing this a bit less could go a long way. Moderation is one thing, but realizing the dire effects of alcohol and social gatherings as "stress-relieving" activities is another. Finding a release solely in alcohol, substances, or social charms does help you blow off steam once in a while, and studies even show that *careful* choices and infrequent alcohol consumption can have sporadic health benefits.

But think of it this way—each time you do that, you might be taking 2 steps forward for your stress levels, but in terms of digestion and overall health you're taking 5 steps backwards. Moderate consumption does show benefits, but that does *NOT* mean that starting to drink alcohol means you will be healthier. Rather, consumption leads you to walking a very fine line, and can always lead to heavier amounts that disrupt digestion.

With that being said—long story short, turn to other methods or forms of stress-relief in your life, beyond alcohol consumption or partying (of course, if you don't do that, you're in the clear!). If you're doing this excessively, find other ways to blow off steam. Alcohol has been shown to disrupt practically every element of the digestive system, even damaging the lining of the stomach, creating acid reflux, inflaming the intestines and even leading to mouth or GI cancers. Again—while it might make you feel great in the short term, too much can be disparaging to health in the long term.

Rest, Relax... and Take Your Time!

Last but not least: take your time. Sit-down meals are starting to become a thing of the past in this modern, hustle-and-bustle world, while eating out at restaurants with highly rich, harmful foods is starting to take over. This loss is highly lamentable, and the only way this can be different is through a huge lifestyle change.

Many argue that our loss of appreciation and ritual for the sit-down meal has robbed us of one of gut health's most important elements: giving importance to food and digestion in the first place. Cooking whole foods at home, moreover, is cheaper and healthier than restaurant meals or grabbing processed foods at gas stations, as the result of having little time to eat! But as modern jobs and lives are getting busier and busier, eating and health are becoming less of a priority. Of course, this leads to poor gut health.

Cultures around the world place a lot of emphasis on "rest and digest," and relaxing times reserved for after meals. Working that into your life, and making that a belief or even a mantra, might be difficult at first; especially if you're used to grabbing on-the-go meals or have way too many daily demands.

But who knows—maybe by placing a renewed importance on cooking, sitting down, and even connecting to others over food, we can all rekindle an important connection to our digestive health and great foods: a connection that has long been lost, perhaps even at the expense of our own health.

THANK YOU

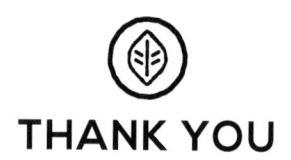

I'd like to thank you, again, for purchasing this book and exploring all the ins-and-outs of digestive health with me. I hope that my knowledge, research, and journey have given you some invaluable ideas and tips you can use to inform your own unique path—a path towards prime gut health, healthy eating, and the energy and wellness you so deserve!

When you do feel lost in the intricate, but confusing world of digestive health, you can always turn to this book again. Review the many foods to focus on, to get you back on track. Take a second look at those foods you should be steering clear of, or even give yourself a primer on the vitamins, minerals, macronutrients and even lifestyle changes you could implement to stay within the lines.

Maybe another glimpse at potential probiotics for your diet will help re-motivate you again, and of course: never forget to peruse the many healthful, healing herbs that could steer you towards the right track once more! Remember to use them cautiously and in an informed way. Knowledge and self-education is power, and if you are ever in doubt about your gut health, symptoms you're experiencing or making changes to your diet—never hesitate to contact a professional health practitioner who can help you with those issues.

I will leave you here, but stay connected and in touch with the *Carma Books* community and email list for more books on holistic, natural, and plant-based health. Reach out again soon for forthcoming, much-talked-about health subjects, just like *Healthy Gut Solution*, along with plenty of experiences and sharing of tips and knowledge on how to empower healing in your own life—and to get the most mileage out of your health potential!

Until next time, I wish you a wonderful, beautiful journey of your own, in happiness and health.

A WORD FROM THE PUBLISHER

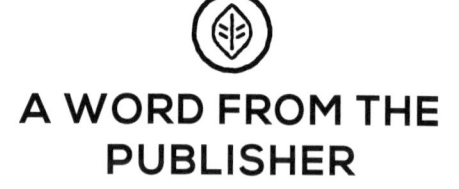

Hi, I'm Carmen, a holistic health geek with a passion for health, herbalism, natural remedies, as well as whole-food and plant-based lifestyles. After resolving various health issues I have struggled with for many years, I aim to inspire and help improve your health and longevity by sharing the tireless hours of research and valuable information I have discovered throughout my journey. Through the power of nutrition and lifestyle, with an evidence-based approach, I believe you can achieve your health and wellness goals.

If you enjoyed this book, I would love to hear how it has benefited you and invite you to leave a short review on Amazon - your valuable feedback is always appreciated!

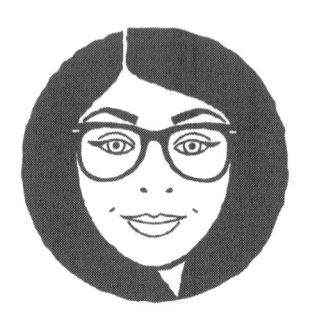

♡

*You are invited to to join our **Free Book Club** mailing list. Sign up via our website to receive **special offers** and **free for a limited time** Health & Wellness eBooks!*

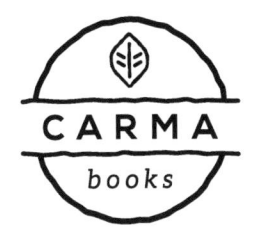

CARMA
books

'A conscious approach to health & wellness'

carmabooks.com

THANK YOU

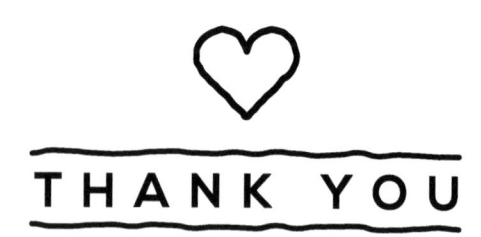